Chair Based Resistance Exercises for Seniors

Strengthening Exercises for Silver Citizens

Dr. Monica Haman

Other Books by This Author

https://www.amazon.com/dp/B0BT9912YX

https://www.amazon.com/dp/B0BX2FRN1Q

https://www.amazon.com/dp/B0BRX25GC6

https://www.amazon.com/dp/B0BSTMZ7PJ

https://www.amazon.com/dp/B0BRDGMMRB

https://www.amazon.com/dp/B0BRDGMMRB

https://www.amazon.com/dp/B0CMPMCG97

TABLE OF CONTENTS

INTRODUCTION

There are many who would have you believe that our greatest achievements are behind us, but I am here to announce that such talk is false. Based on my own life, I firmly believe that the passing years only add richness and meaning to the tapestry that is life. Others may say that as you become older, you have to slow down and give up your vitality, but I'm here to prove them wrong.

Yes, my friend, you can feel better than ever, and it all starts with a simple choice: a choice to invest in your well-being, beginning exactly where you are, even if that's in the comfort of a chair. If you've lost touch with your inner power, flexibility, and the inexhaustible joy of movement, this book is here to help you find your way back.

If you choose to follow my lead, I will guide you through each stimulating chapter, revealing the wonders of resistance band workouts from sitting leg exercises to gentle tricep extensions. Envision waking up to a new sense of purpose, a day full of vitality, and your soul moving to the beat of a life well-lived.

This is more than a book; it's a call to action to live life to the fullest, even in our twilight years, by rejecting conventional wisdom and making the most of every opportunity. Let this be a tribute to your fortitude, a proclamation that age is not a barrier but a blank slate upon which we can create the masterpiece of our lives.

Come along with me on this incredible adventure and celebrate the thrill of living to the fullest with me, no matter how old you are. Within these pages is your ticket to a thrilling new experience.

With love and support,

Dr. Monica Haman

Chapter One

Understanding Resistance Bands

Hello and welcome to the essence of renewal. Within these simple resistance bands, a world of possibility awaits us, the wise and magnificent elders. Let us take a journey into the center of power and energy together.

Understanding How Senior Bands Work

Resistance bands provide a calibrated challenge, providing moderate but effective muscle engagement.

Muscle Activation: These bands simultaneously engage several muscle areas, enabling balanced strength growth.

Moderate Advancement: Because of their adaptability, they allow for moderate advancement, allowing us to raise intensity at our own pace.

Why Resistance Bands are Ideal for Senior Citizens

1.) Adjustable Resistance: Bands are available in a variety of tensions, allowing for customisation based on individual strength levels.

2.) Reduced Joint Impact: Unlike heavyweights, bands provide resistance without causing joint stress, making them perfect for elders.

3.) Bands cater to a wide range of movements, from seated exercises to standing stretches, developing general flexibility.

Simple Techniques for Safety

1.) Warm-up properly: Begin with mild motions to warm up muscles and prepare them for resistance.

2.) Hold the bands with an open hand, preventing excessive tension on the fingers and wrists.

3.) Maintain a solid posture throughout workouts, utilizing the core for balance and support.

4.) Smooth Movements: Execute movements slowly and steadily, focusing on controlled muscle contractions.

5.) Breathing Rhythm: Match your breathing to your actions, expelling during effort and inhaling during relaxation.

6.) Avoid Overstretching: Avoid overstretching by utilizing bands of adequate resistance to engage muscles without strain.

7.) Take frequent rests between exercises to reduce muscle exhaustion and allow muscles to recuperate.

8.) Consultation: If you are unsure about specific activities, get professional advice to ensure a safe and individualized fitness plan.

9.) Cool down by wrapping up exercises with moderate stretches that promote muscle relaxation and flexibility.

Accept these subtleties, my friends, for they are the keepers of our safety and the architects of our growth. With these ideas, we embark on a journey of wisdom and care for our bodies, not only physical transformation. Are you ready to go into the depths of this knowledge? Let us delve into the complexities of resistance bands, making sure that every movement contributes to our collective well-being.

Chapter Two

Strong Legs with Bands

Ah, the foundation of our mobility and grace – our legs. In this chapter, we dive deep into the art of strengthening these pillars of vitality using the subtle yet potent resistance bands. Join me as we explore a world of gentle yet effective leg exercises designed specifically for the seasoned souls among us.

Seated Leg Exercises: Building Lower Body Strength

1.) Chair Leg Lifts: To build strength and stability, lift one leg at a time while using your quadriceps and calves.

2.) Seated Leg Press: To increase lower body power, press your legs up against the band's resistance, focusing on your glutes and thighs.

3.) Ankle Rolls: To increase flexibility and encourage ankle joint mobility, rotate your ankles in a circular manner.

Chair Squats: Toning Thighs and Hips

1.) Seated Squats: Squat while seated to engage your thighs and hips and build endurance and muscular tone.

2.) Chair Side Leg Lifts: While seated, raise your legs sideways to target your hips and outer thighs and to improve the definition of your muscles.

Leg Stretches: Improving Leg Flexibility with Bands

1.) Seated Forward Bend: To increase hamstring flexibility, extend your legs forward while seated with the use of bands for more resistance.

2.) Seated Inner Thigh Stretch: To stretch your inner thighs and increase flexibility and mobility, spread your legs wide and press against the band.

3.) Stretch your quadriceps and hip flexors by standing and pulling one foot toward your glutes using bands.

Allow these exercises to create a movement symphony, gradually returning strength and flexibility to our legs. Remember, my dear friends, that every stretch and lift is a thank you to these amazing limbs that carry us through life's experiences.

We're not simply toning muscles with each exercise; we're also fostering the very essence of our mobility and independence. Are you ready to embark on this life-changing leg journey? Let's take

things slowly at first.

Chapter Three

Arm and Upper Body Strength

Our arms, the extensions of our emotions, the instruments of our everyday victories. This chapter will reveal the keys of improving the strength of these cherished limbs. As we age gracefully, it becomes increasingly important to preserve the energy in our upper bodies, allowing us to embrace life's delights with ease and confidence.

Easy Arm Lifts: Strengthening Arm Muscles

1.) Seated Bicep Curls: Raise bands toward shoulders to contract biceps and enhance arm tone and strength.

2.) Tricep Extensions: To target the triceps and improve upper arm stiffness, extend your arms overhead and then bend your elbows behind your head.

3.) Exercises for Wrist Flexors and Extensors: Promote wrist flexibility and avoid joint stiffness by using bands as resistance.

Band Rows for Upper Back: Improving Posture

1.) Seated Band Rows: Pull bands toward chest to target upper back muscles, improve posture, and stabilize shoulders.

2.) Back extensions: While lying prone, raise your arms and chest against resistance from a band to strengthen your upper back and improve the support of your spine.

Gentle Tricep Extensions: Toning Arm Flab

1.) Seated Tricep Dips: While seated, press your palms on the seat, raise and lower your body, contract your triceps, and define your arms.

2.) Standing Tricep Kickbacks: To tone your triceps and improve the shape of your arms, stand and stretch your arms backward against band resistance.

In these exercises, we find the grace to lift our arms with confidence as well as strength. Every curl and extension becomes a monument to the years of wisdom carried by our arms. They are a tribute to our resiliency, and with each movement, we are shaping our ability to reach out and embrace the world, not just muscles.

Chapter Four

Balance and Core Stability

Let's talk about something incredible: core strength and balance. This shift was noticeable not in a grandiose moment, but in the modest successes of everyday life. Consider this: I was reaching for a high shelf in my kitchen, which used to make me nervous. This time, however, I felt anchored, confident, and steady. It was as if my body had discovered a new harmony, a balance it hadn't felt in years.

Bending to pick up items from the floor felt less intimidating. My core muscles supported my movements, making me feel agile and in command.Sitting up straight had nearly become instinctive. The mild heat in my core muscles reminded me that they were becoming stronger, effortlessly supporting my spine, and in so many other ways.

These workouts are more than just routines; they are a gateway to a more confident, balanced you. They make everyday activities into occasions to celebrate your newfound strength. As we begin this chapter together, imagine these practical scenarios becoming triumphant moments not only for me, but also for you.

Seated Balance Activities: Enhancing Stability

1.) Chair Leg Raises: Raise one leg at a time while focusing on your core, feeling the band's gentle tug. This will increase your leg strength and stability.

2.) Torso Twists in a Seated Position: Gently twist while seated, sensing the resistance against your motions, using your core muscles, and enhancing your balance and flexibility.

3.) Chair Yoga Poses: Sit with bands to support yourself as you embrace the peaceful silence of yoga. Feel the strength of this pose pour through your core, nourishing your equilibrium and mental clarity.Core Strengthening with Bands: Gentle Ab Workouts

4.) Seated Russian Twists: This exercise will tone your oblique muscles, slim your waist, and strengthen your core as you twist your torso back and forth while gripping the band.

5.) Leg Raises with Bands: While sitting, raise your legs and feel the engagement in your lower abdomen. This exercise tones your core and improves pelvic stability. You can use bands for resistance.

6.) Pelvic tilts: While seated, gently tilt your pelvis by pressing on the band and feeling the muscles in your lower back and core contract in unison to strengthen and stabilize your spine.

Chapter Five

Flexibility and Comfort

Picture this: you wake up, the world still wrapped in the quiet embrace of dawn. As you stretch, you feel the gentle pull of the resistance band, and suddenly, your body awakens like a flower unfolding its petals to the sun. In this chapter, we delve into the realm of flexibility and comfort, exploring the myriad ways these bands can transform your mornings and infuse your entire day with a sense of vitality.

Stretching with Bands: Increasing Overall Flexibility

Morning Band Stretch Routine:

1.) Reach Above: Take a tall stance, hold the band in your hands, and extend your arm above. Your arms and spine will both feel stretched, energising your entire upper body.

2.) Stretch your lower back and hamstrings while sitting in a seated forward bend. Loop the band around your feet and lean forward, feeling the slight resistance.

3.) Lateral Side Stretch: Hold the band in one hand, stand with your feet hip-width apart, and extend sideways. Savor the satisfying tug along your side that expands your rib cage and increases the flexibility of your spine.

4.) Dynamic Leg Swings: Swing your legs back and forth while maintaining your balance by holding the band. To make sure your legs are prepared for the trials of the day, feel your hip flexors and hamstrings waking up.

Neck and Shoulder Relaxation: Easing Stiffness

1.) Morning Neck and Shoulders Release: Take a comfortable seat, wrap the band over one hand, and pull it gently to the side. Experience the calming stretch that eases stress and encourages relaxation throughout your neck.

2.) Shoulder Opener: Raise your arms while standing or sitting with the band behind your back and both ends grasped. Feel the tension in your shoulders release as they become more mobile.

3.) Ear-to-Shoulder-Stretch: Stretch your ear to your shoulder by sitting up straight, holding one end of the band, and cocking your head to the side so that your ear is gently guided toward your shoulder. Enjoy the stretch along your neck as any stiffness from the previous night melts away.

Gentle Hip Movements: Enhancing Mobility

1.) Morning Hip Awakening: Grasp the band around your ankles, place your hands on your hips, and move your hips in a circular motion to awaken your hips in the morning. Feel the mild resistance as it improves hip range of motion and gets your lower body ready for the day's activities.

2.) Seated Hip Opener: Cross-legged, wrap the band around your thighs, and push outward against the resistance to perform the seated hip opener. Feel the tension after a restful night go as your hips expand.

3.) Dynamic Hip Flexor Stretch: With the band wrapped around your front foot, bend at the knee. To ensure your hips are prepared for activity, gently lean forward and feel the band give your hip flexors a thorough stretch.

With these morning stretches, your body becomes a flexible and comfortable canvas, ready to welcome the day's experiences. Each movement is more than just a stretch; it's a gift to your body, a self-care routine that sets the tone for a day full of ease and vitality.

Are you ready to make every morning a celebration of comfort and flexibility? Let's get started with these exercises, waking up your body with each gentle tug of the band to ensure your days begin with grace and flexibility.

Chapter Six

Light Cardio and Relaxation

The song of the breath, the rhythm of the heart - this chapter is all about infusing your days with mild cardio and the serene embrace of relaxation. Consider beginning your day with the liveliness of a modest cardio session, your heart dancing to a beat that is invigorating but not overwhelming. Then, when the day comes to an end, imagine yourself slipping into a realm of serenity and tranquility, your body and mind finding consolation in the soft caress of relaxation techniques.

Seated Marching: Simple Cardio for Seniors

1.) Morning Cardio Boost: March in place while sitting up straight with the band under your feet. Sitting comfortably in a chair, feel your heart rate gradually increase, your muscles waking, and your whole body becoming filled with life.

2.) Increased Heart Rate: Enjoy the pleasant increase in heart rate that comes with each deliberate movement. This promotes cardiovascular health without the strain of high-impact activities.

3.) Enhanced Energy: Take note of how this morning routine gives you a boost of energy that enables you to tackle the day with renewed strength and endurance for all of your everyday tasks.

Breathing Exercises: Relaxation and Stress Relief

1.) Deep Breathing: Position the band across your belly while sitting or lying down. Breathe in deeply, pushing against the band with your diaphragm, and then release the breath gradually. With each breath, feel your body relax and stress melt away, bringing you a sense of inner peace and tranquility.

2.) Stress-Free Breaths: Visualize letting go of all your cares and anxieties for the day with each exhale. Imagine your spirit light and your intellect clear as your breath lifts the weights.

3.) Mindful Pause: The goal of this practice is to relax the mind as much as the body. Breathe deeply and allow your mind to calm down like a pond after a rainstorm, embracing a peaceful moment amidst the craziness of life.

Band Meditation: Calmness and Peace of Mind

1.) Guided Meditation: Sit comfortably with the band loosely in your hands throughout the guided meditation. Shut your eyes and concentrate on your respiration. Imagine drawing in peace with each inhale and releasing stress with each exhale. The band becomes into an anchor that keeps you rooted in the here and now.

2.) Visualizing Relaxation: Imagine yourself somewhere serene—a forest, a beach, or any other location that makes you feel at ease. Feel the band as a physical representation of your serenity, connecting your inner and outer peace as you hold it.

3.) Body and Mind Harmony: Feel how your body and mind are one, with the band serving as a metaphor for the link between them. Allow the band to serve as a constant reminder of your inner fortitude and capacity to remain composed in the face of adversity as you meditate.

I recognize that cardiac exercises aren't for everyone, especially as we become older. But here's a little secret: they're the unsung heroes of our well-being. Cardiovascular health is more than just getting our hearts to beat quicker; it is also about getting them to beat stronger and more efficiently. I get that it may not be the most glamorous aspect of our exercise program, but it is absolutely necessary. It's like giving our hearts a daily injection of vitality, allowing them to easily pump life through our veins.

It's a bet on our future, a guarantee of a healthier, more active tomorrow. So, rather than viewing it as an onerous duty, consider it a wonderful present we give to ourselves: the gift of a vibrant, resilient heart and a body capable of keeping up with all the experiences life has in store for us. Embrace cardio out of love for the beautiful vessel that carries us through life, not out of necessity.

Chapter Seven

Bands in Everyday Life

Consider your morning routine, which was formerly dull but has now been imbued with the colorful energy of resistance bands. Imagine yourself in nature, the rustling leaves harmonizing with the stretch of your band, and feel the joy of being connected to the world around you. Consider the laughter and joint efforts that occur during family band sessions, where love and health interweave to form a link that extends beyond physical workouts.

Integrating Bands into Daily Life: A Symphony of Wellness

1.) Morning Band Ritual: Stretch your arms with the band as the world awakens, welcoming the day with vigor and purpose. Allow this morning routine to serve as your daily affirmation, a subtle signal to your body that you're prepared to face any challenge.

2.) Band-Aided Exercises: Transform the ordinary into the remarkable. Allow the resistance band to be your companion while you sweep, vacuum, or arrange. Experience a burn in your muscles as you transform household tasks into short exercises that demonstrate your perseverance and strength.

3.) Band Adventures in Nature: Play live with your band. Stretch it while encircling a tree to experience the oneness of your physical form with the environment. Let the birds be your supporters, the wind your friend, and the band your link to a more profound relationship with the natural world.

Shared Fitness, Shared Joy: Building Bonds Through Bands

1.) Family Band Evenings: Get your loved ones together for family band nights. Experience the thrill of passing the band, a representation of harmony and well-being among all, from one hand to the next. You're strengthening the ties that bind your family together at these times in addition to your physical health.

2.) Fitness and Friendships: Get your mates together for a band practice. Find emotional support as well as physical strength in the laughing and companionship. Let the teamwork serve as evidence of the strength of friendship, transforming casual get-togethers into occasions to celebrate one another's health and unity.

Dear reader, as we near the finish of this journey together, I want you to know that this chapter isn't simply the end; it's also the beginning. It's an invitation to a life where fitness isn't a chore but a joy, where every movement is a dance, every stretch a song, and every shared activity a symphony of community. May your days be filled with unlimited energy, your heart with unshakable strength, and your spirit with enduring joy as you enjoy these everyday moments of wellness. Here's to you, to us, and to the lovely, healthy lives we're creating.

As you move forward, remember that every step, no matter how tiny, is a win. With a grateful heart and a proud spirit, I wish you not only good health but also abundant happiness and the strength to continue this magnificent journey of well-being. Here's to the incredible life that lies ahead of you, full of vigor, love, and limitless possibilities.

9 798867 583149